Your Key to Broad Shoulders
Revised Edition

Written and Published by Bill Pearl
Edited by George and Tuesday Coates
Layout and Illustrations by Richard R. Thornley Jr.

Bill Pearl
P.O. Box 1080
Phoenix, Oregon 97535
Email: support@billpearl.com
Website: www.billpearl.com

ISBN-13: 978-1-938855-11-5

Notice of Rights

Medical Disclaimer - See Your Doctor

Most people may do all of the exercises found in this book with no ill effects. However, if certain movements cause discomfort they should be eliminated. See your doctor and get the doctor's approval on the total fitness program.

Table of Contents

Chapter 1

Introduction

Broad shoulders are admired and sought by everyone interested in body-building. Deep broad shoulders are a symbol of strength and masculinity. Ever since man became interested in physical culture, he has desired to enhance his appearance with strong broad shoulders.

One does not have to be born with a wide shoulder girdle to possess them. Hard work and sensible training will develop large shoulder muscles. I know two of the all-time greats, who structurally did not have broad shoulders, but through concentrated training, they created for themselves wide shoulders and won top place in the strength and physique world.

Bill Pearl is one who has excellent skeletal structure and possesses extremely wide shoulders, but he has worked to increase their width and depth by the exercises and courses outlined on the following pages.

Do not improvise. Follow closely the recommended way to do each exercise. You can improve. Give forth the effort and reap the fruits of your work.

Good Luck!
Leo Stern

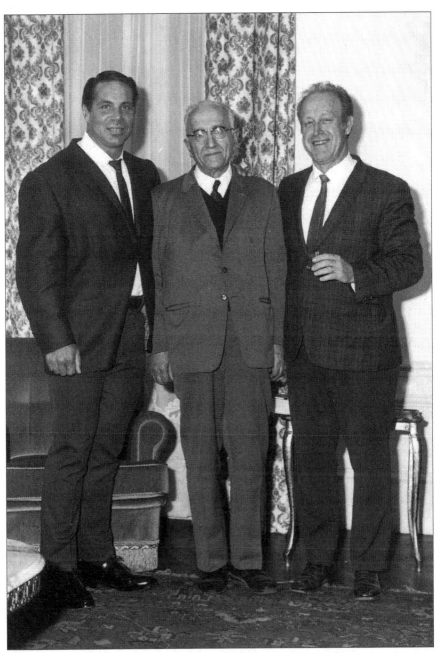

Bill Pearl with two of the finest modern day physique photographers: Gregor Arax, of Paris, France, and Leo Stern, of San Diego, California. For nearly 50 years, Arax photographed the major European contests, including the NABBA "Mr. Universe."

Chapter 2

Building Broad Shoulders

Broad shoulders are something that can add as much to a person's physical appearance as any other part of the anatomy. Regardless of how the person is dressed, broad shoulders are hard to hide and will automatically, even if subconsciously, make an impression on any person who is interested in the physical aspects of the human body.

Throughout the years that I have acted as an instructor in health studios and the many years I have spent training myself, I can say that it is much easier for most people to talk about someone with broad shoulders than it is to build a set for themselves. I have also found that very few people really know exactly what to do to improve their shoulders, except for a few standard exercises.

The width of the shoulders is generally governed by the length of the clavicle bones. If you are fortunate to have exceptionally long clavicles, your shoulders will be broader than normal and the progress will be even more impressive.

We cannot concern ourselves too much about how long or how short a person's clavicle bones are. A person can still improve his shoulder width by proper weight training and this is the reason for writing this book.

This book is designed to help you improve the shoulders as quickly and completely as it is possibly known today. We have not left out any muscle group and have concerned ourselves with the small muscles as well as the large muscle groups of the shoulders.

I strongly suggest that you follow the courses outlined as they are written. Do not deviate from them, if at all possible. All of the courses are written exactly as we feel they should be done and are placed as they are for a particular reason. If you find that one exercise seems to bother your shoulders, I suggest you stop the exercise and supplement it with another that does not bother you.

Concentration while you are doing an exercise is extremely important and will speed the progress of the muscle. Be sure that you do not get in the habit of handling too much weight as to do the exercise improperly. Always train within your limits. Keep a positive attitude towards your workouts and think even more positively about the muscle group that you are trying to bring along a little faster and you will be sure to show remarkable improvement. Train hard and be consistent.

Best of Luck,
Bill Pearl

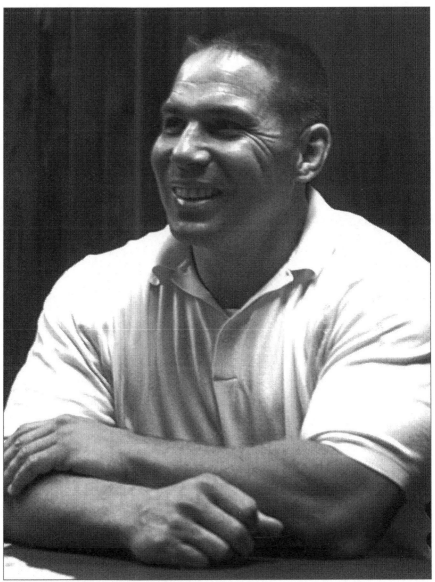

Bill Pearl smiling after a good days work.

Chapter 3

How to Use this Book

If a person is interested in weight training for more than basic conditioning, it is imperative that he study each illustration and description before attempting a new exercise. Progress definitely can be deterred if an exercise is done incorrectly.

Many exercises can be accomplished with the exact same motion but will affect different areas of a muscle by the angle at which the exercise is performed. For example: an exercise done on a flat bench, or an incline bench, will put different emphasis on the same muscle even though the same motion, weight and equipment are used.

It is therefore necessary to perform exercises from as many different angles that are reasonable and to use as many variations that are reasonable to develop a fully matured muscular physique.

On the following pages, highly accurate drawings appear that will enable you to see the pieces of equipment used to perform each exercise and the style used for each movement. Each exercise includes the proper name of the exercise, the muscle group most affected, "degree of difficulty" information, and a written description of how the exercise should be done.

The "degree of difficulty" information appearing below each exercise heading will give you at a glance what exercise may be suited for your present physical condition.

NOTE: It is not necessarily true that an exercise considered "easy" may not be just as effective as one considered "hard". Any exercise can be made more or less difficult, depending on the weight used or the effort put forth.

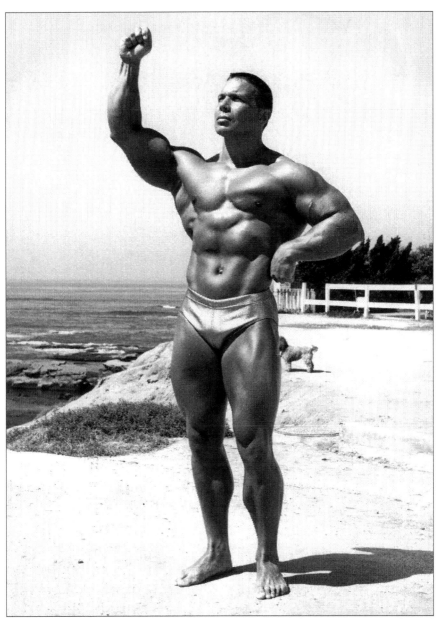

At this stage of Pearl's bodybuilding career, he had changed to a lacto-ovo-vegetarian diet and was still able to maintain his massive size. His shoulders, in particular, were at their career widest.

Chapter 4

Training Advice

Training Advice

Shoulders can he developed. Even though one does not have the bone structure for broad shoulders, muscles can be developed to broaden and give the desired width to your shoulders. If you are fortunate enough to have the natural wide shoulders, which every bodybuilder desires, you can still improve them by working these exercises along with your regular training program. If you are going to specialize, do the schedules outlined at the beginning of your workout schedule and then continue with the balance of the exercises, working your arms, chest, midsection, and legs.

It is possible to improve your shoulders and continue with your over-all body workout. To get the most from this type of program, use it at the beginning of the program and emphasize strict adherence to the instructions. Do not get sloppy on the execution of the exercises. Anything worth doing is worth doing right. Use the prescribed series for at least a period of six weeks and then change and work on series 2-3-4-5. When you are in a balanced condition, work on any weak portion of the deltoid that you feel requires improvement.

It is best to start with the basic movements, and then advance to the more difficult forms of shoulder or deltoid work. Bear in mind we are only interested in muscle and nothing else.

Training Hints

Remember, you must analyze for yourself and decide which part of your deltoid needs the most work, and then reduce the sets on the strong or better developed part. Add more sets to the weak part of the deltoid. There is a limit and when excessive sets are done the muscle does not grow, so there is a normal and reasonable amount of work to bring about the best results. To eliminate confusion, follow this procedure. Do not add sets if the back part of your deltoid is weak and the side is not. Instead of doing five sets of an exercise for building the side portion of the deltoid, cut it down to two to three sets and work harder on the exercises which work and build the rear

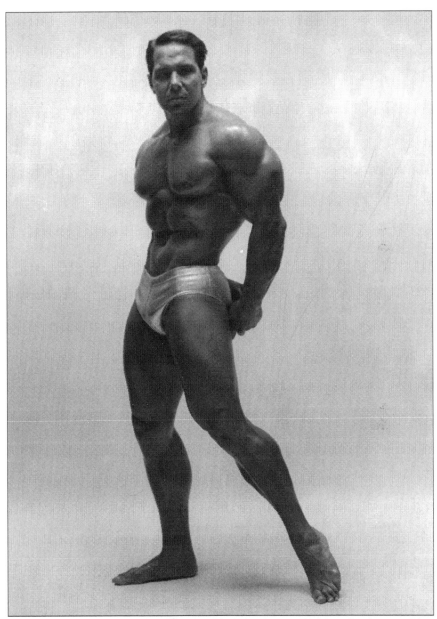

Bill had the largest muscular arm in the world for several years. It measured an honest cold 20 3/8 inches at a bodyweight of 218 pounds.

deltoid. Now, as stated before, over-working a muscle will tend to hold its growth back. It is a matter of the muscle never being able to fully recuperate and build in size and strength.

One must find the normal output for themselves. We have given you what we feel is the right number of sets and you can either increase or reduce the amount, whichever fits your particular physical makeup.

Shoulder Injury Rehabilitation and Prevention of Reinjury

This part is important to you who have suffered a shoulder dislocation or shoulder separation. There are exercises you must do to build the shoulder back to normal and exercises you should never do. Now, we will briefly describe and illustrate the shoulder joint, so you can better understand the problem.

The shoulder girdle is made of the collar bone (clavicle) and the shoulder blade (scapula). The clavicle articulates with the sternum, but the scapula has no boney attachment. The clavicle bone has important muscle attachments that give support to the shoulder joint. Examine the drawings describing the shoulder joint.

When an injury occurs, either a muscle or ligament is pulled or torn. When this happens the humerus bone is pulled out of the ball socket cavity of the scapula. Rest is necessary and one should never resume weight training until his doctor gives permission.

Always start with light weights and use restricted exercises that are controlled. Do not stretch or pull the shoulder. Never do straight arm pullovers or bent arm pullovers, chins or others of this nature until the shoulder is back to normal.

The exercises to use in restoring the shoulder to normal are: (1) close grip military press, keeping a tension on the muscles at all times. Do not stretch out overhead, but make a complete extension and lockout the elbows. (2) Regular barbell rowing motion with a narrow grip (shoulder width). Do not attempt to handle a heavy poundage. Allow the barbell to extend to arm's length, keeping tension on the bar all the while. Keep the shoulders in a firm rigid position. (3) The prone press with a close grip, no wider than shoulders' width. Again use a light poundage. Try to keep the muscle under tension all the time you are doing your repetitions. Use a slow even rhythm when doing these exercises and have complete control over the movement of the barbell.

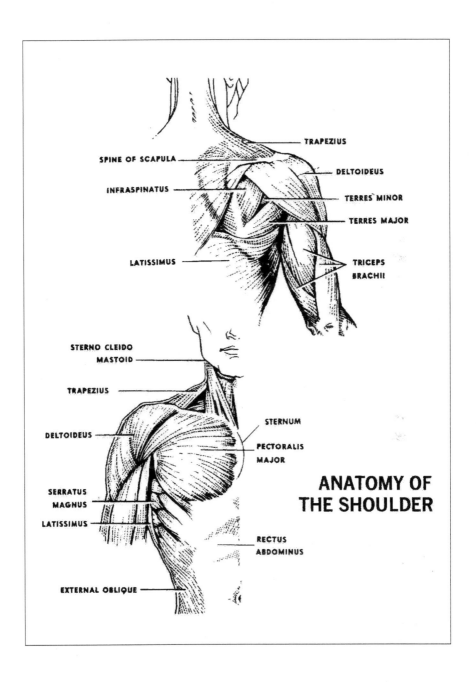

TRAPEZIUS

SPINE OF SCAPULA

DELTOIDEUS

INFRASPINATUS

TERRES MINOR

TERRES MAJOR

LATISSIMUS

TRICEPS
BRACHII

STERNO CLEIDO
MASTOID

TRAPEZIUS

STERNUM

DELTOIDEUS

PECTORALIS
MAJOR

SERRATUS
MAGNUS

LATISSIMUS

ANATOMY OF
THE SHOULDER

RECTUS
ABDOMINUS

EXTERNAL OBLIQUE

SKELETAL STRUCTURE OF THE SHOULDER

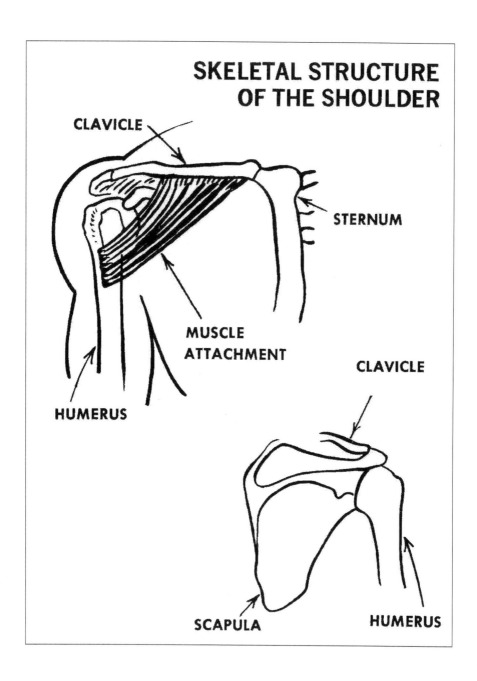

CLAVICLE

STERNUM

MUSCLE ATTACHMENT

HUMERUS

CLAVICLE

SCAPULA

HUMERUS

This page has been intentionally left blank.

Chapter 5

Equipment Needed

Equipment needed to perform the exercises in this training guide.

- Barbell
- Dumbbells
- Flat Bench
- Incline Bench
- Chair
- Stool

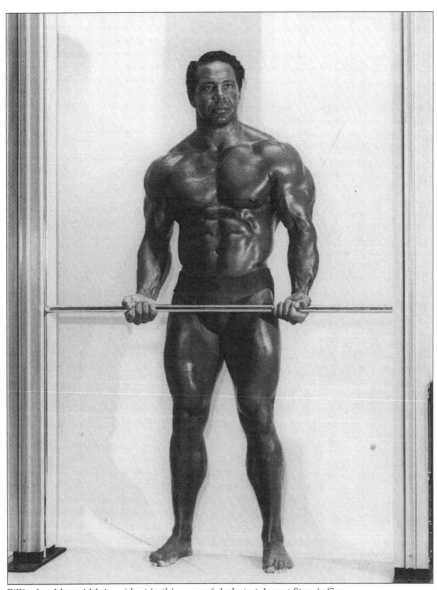

Bill's shoulder width is evident in this powerful photo taken at Stern's Gym.

Chapter 6

Course One

The following courses are for individuals who have been training for a period of years. Beginners should do only one set of each exercise on course one. After completing the six week period, start course two and do two sets of each exercise. Do not do more than three sets of each exercise until you have been working out for a year or more. Work within your own limit

EXERCISES:

1. Standing Military Press	3 sets of 8-10
2. Medium Grip Barbell Upright Rowing	3 sets of 8-10
3. Seated Back Supported Palms in Dumbbell Press	3 sets of 8
4. Bent Over Head Supported Dumbbell Rear Deltoid Raise	3 sets of 8

- Follow this course of exercises for a six week period
- Do Three Workouts per Week

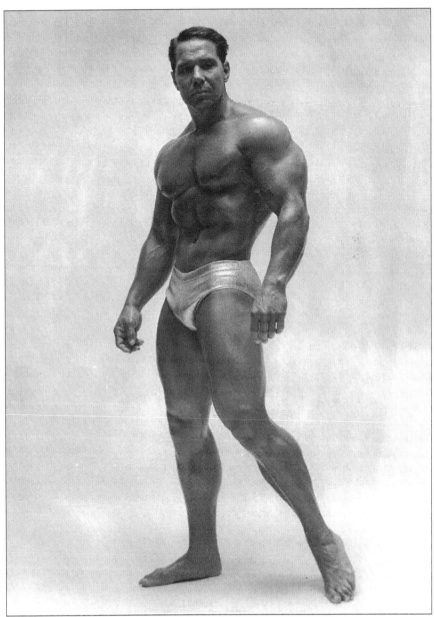

A five foot measuring tape was not large enough to measure Pearl's shoulder girth at the time this photo was taken.

STANDING MILITARY PRESS

Muscle Group: Front and outer deltoids
Degree of Difficulty: Intermediate

This is the standard military press. Clean the weight to the chest. Lock the legs and hips solidly. This will give you a solid platform from which to push. Keep the elbows in slightly and under the bar, press the weight overhead, lock the arms out. When lowering the barbell to the upper chest, be sure it rests on the chest and is not held with the arms. If the chest is held high, it will give you a nice shelf on which to place the barbell and to push from. Inhale before the press and exhale when lowering the barbell.

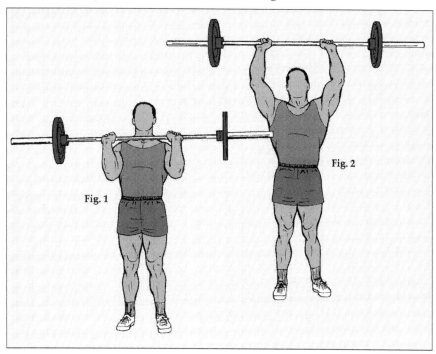

Fig. 1

Fig. 2

MEDIUM GRIP BARBELL UPRIGHT ROWING

Muscle Group: Front deltoids and trapezius
Degree of Difficulty: Intermediate

Place your hands on a barbell with the palms facing down and use a hand grip about eighteen inches apart. With the barbell at arm's length while you are standing erect and in a stationary position, pull the weight straight up until it is nearly under the chin. Keep the elbows out to the sides and in the top position the elbows are nearly as high as your ears. Keep the barbell in close to the body and pause momentarily at the top before letting the weight back to starting position. Inhale as you raise the bar and exhale as you lower the bar.

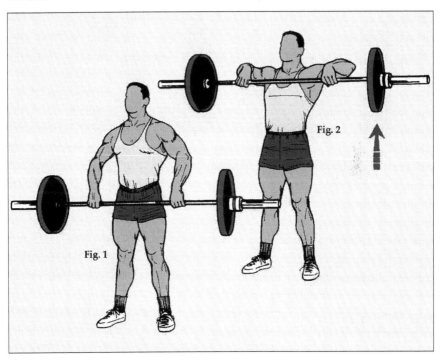

Fig. 2

Fig. 1

SEATED BACK SUPPORTED PALMS IN DUMBBELL PRESS

Muscle Group: Front and outer deltoids
Degree of Difficulty: Intermediate

Clean two dumbbells to your shoulders and then sit on a bench or chair that will give support to your upper back. Keep your feet planted firmly on the floor. With the palms facing inward, inhale and press the dumbbells to arm's length overhead. Exhale as you are lowering the weights back to starting position. Be sure to keep the arms in as you are performing this exercise. Do not let the elbows wander out.

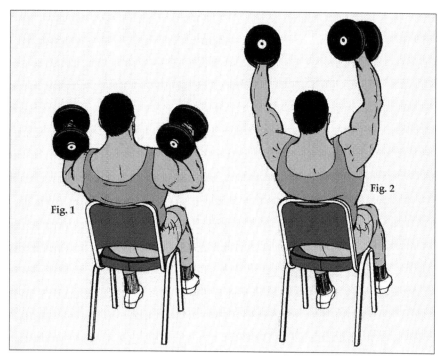

Fig. 1

Fig. 2

BENT OVER HEAD SUPPORTED DUMBBELL REAR DELTOID RAISE

Muscle Group: Rear deltoids
Degree of Difficulty: Difficult

Bend over and support your forehead on a comfortable object that is not quite waist high. Lock the elbows and keep the arms straight. Bring the dumbbells to the position shown in illustration #2, hold for a short period and contract the rear deltoid muscles. Do not swing the dumbbells up, keep the body rigid and head resting on the object. Do the work with the rear deltoids and muscles of the upper back. Be sure to bring the dumbbells straight out to the sides and make an effort to keep the hands forward in line with your ears at the top position. Inhale up, exhale down.

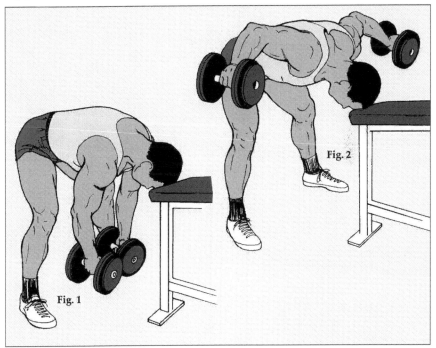

Fig. 1

Fig. 2

Chapter 7

Course Two

The following courses are for individuals who have been training for a period of years. Beginners should do only one set of each exercise on course one. After completing the six week period, start course two and do two sets of each exercise. Do not do more than three sets of each exercise until you have been working out for a year or more. Work within your own limit

EXERCISES:

1. Standing Barbell Press Behind Neck	4 sets of 8-10
2. Wide Grip Bent Over Barbell Rowing	4 sets of 8
3. Seated Palms in Alternated Dumbbell Press	3 sets of 8
4. Standing Medium Grip Front Barbell Raise	3 sets of 8-10

- Follow this course of exercises for a six week period
- Do Three Workouts per Week

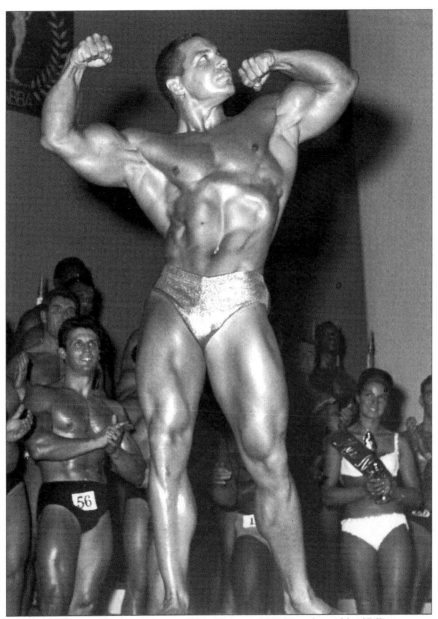

The fruits of labor. Bill Pearl, professional Mr. Universe 1967. Note the width of Bill's shoulders and the taper down to his waist.

STANDING BARBELL PRESS BEHIND NECK

Muscle Group: Front and outer deltoids

Degree of Difficulty: Difficult

Stand with your feet spaced a comfortable distance apart with a barbell placed on your upper back. Use a grip on the bar that is about four to six inches wider than your shoulders. Press the barbell overhead and exhale as you lower the bar to the back of your shoulders. Maintain a solid foundation by keeping the legs straight and the hips flexed. Pause at the shoulders on each repetition before pressing the barbell overhead. Make a full movement of the exercise by touching the barbell to the shoulders each time it is lowered and locking the elbows each time it is pressed overhead.

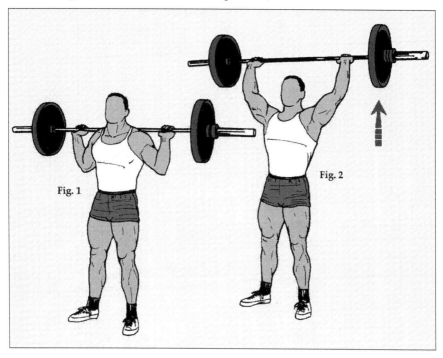

Fig. 1

Fig. 2

WIDE GRIP BENT OVER BARBELL ROWING

Muscle Group: Upper lats
Degree of Difficulty: Intermediate

Place a barbell on the floor in front of you. With your feet about eighteen inches apart, bend down and get a grip on the barbell that is as wide as is comfortably possible. Keep your legs bent and your back parallel to the floor as you inhale and pull the barbell directly up to the lower part of your chest. Do not let the barbell touch the floor once you have begun the exercise. Keep your head up and your back straight.

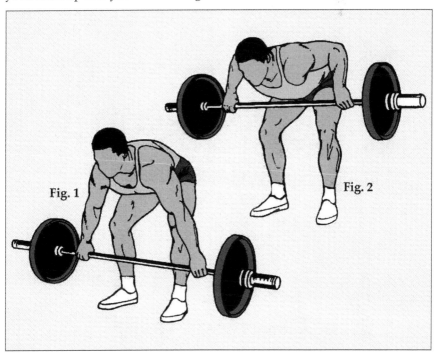

Fig. 1

Fig. 2

SEATED PALMS IN ALTERNATED DUMBBELL PRESS

Muscle Group: Front and outer deltoids

Degree of Difficulty: Intermediate

Clean two dumbbells and sit at the end of a bench. With the dumbbells at shoulder height, commence to press the dumbbell in the right hand to arm's length overhead, keeping the palms in and the elbows and arms in. Lower the dumbbell in the right hand back to starting position and then press the dumbbell in the left hand in the same manner. Maintain a rigid body position, doing all the work with the shoulders and arms. Do not lean from side to side while pressing. Inhale as you start to press the dumbbell and exhale as you are lowering the weight.

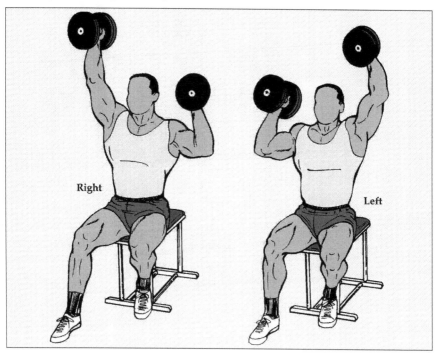

STANDING MEDIUM GRIP FRONT BARBELL RAISE

Muscle Group: Front deltoids
Degree of Difficulty: Intermediate

Use a shoulder width grip on a barbell. Stand with your feet about sixteen inches apart and have the legs and hips in a flexed position to help keep the back straight. With the barbell hanging at arm's length against your upper thighs, inhale and raise the bar straight up, not bending the elbows, until it is directly overhead. Exhale as you are lowering the bar back to starting position. Do not unlock the elbows during the full movement.

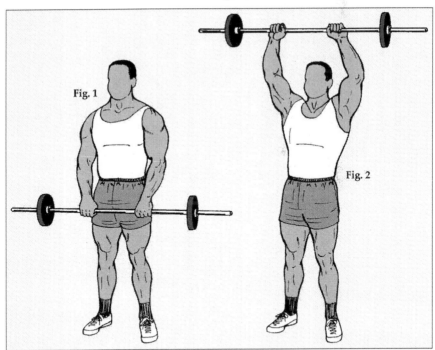

Fig. 1

Fig. 2

Chapter 8

Course Three

The following courses are for individuals who have been training for a period of years. Beginners should do only one set of each exercise on course one. After completing the six week period, start course two and do two sets of each exercise. Do not do more than three sets of each exercise until you have been working out for a year or more. Work within your own limit

EXERCISES:

1. Wide Grip Barbell Upright Rowing	3 sets of 6-8
2. Seated Barbell Press Behind Neck	4 sets of 6-8
3. Standing Cheating Side Lateral Raise	3 sets of 6-8
4. Seated Dumbbell Straight Arm Front Deltoid Raise	3 sets of 8
5. Incline Dumbbell Held to the Front Side Lateral Raise	2 sets of 8-10

- Follow this course of exercises for a six week period
- Do Three Workouts per Week

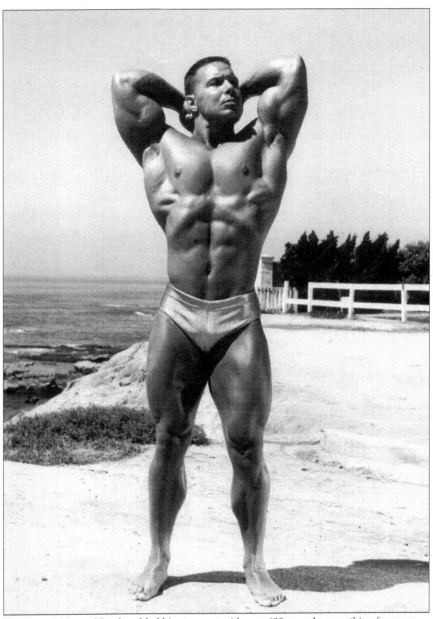

The powerful legs of Pearl enabled him to squat with over 600 pounds, something few men had done prior to 1960.

WIDE GRIP BARBELL UPRIGHT ROWING

Muscle Group: Front deltoids and trapezius
Degree of Difficulty: Difficult

Place your hands on a barbell with your palms facing down and using a grip that is about thirty-two to thirty-six inches apart. With the barbell at arm's length while you are standing erect and in a stationary position, pull the weight straight up until it is nearly under the chin. Keep the elbows out to the sides and in the top position the elbows are nearly as high as your ears. Keep the barbell in close to the body and pause momentarily at the top before letting the weight back to starting position. Inhale as you raise the bar and exhale as you lower the bar.

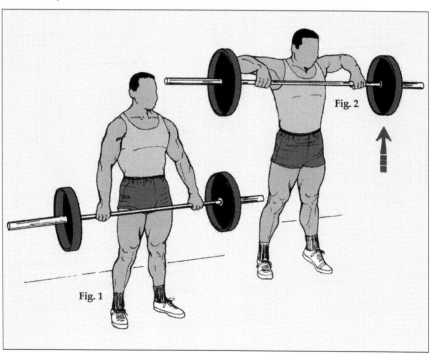

Fig. 1

Fig. 2

SEATED BARBELL PRESS BEHIND NECK

Muscle Group: Front and outer deltoids
Degree of Difficulty: Difficult

Sit at the end of a bench with your feet spaced a comfortable distance apart with a barbell placed on your upper back. Use a grip on the bar that is about four to six inches wider than your shoulders. Keep the elbows directly under the bar. Press the barbell overhead and exhale as you lower the bar to the back of your shoulders. Maintain a solid foundation with your upper body so as not to hyper extend any more than is necessary. Pause at the shoulders on each repetition before pressing the barbell overhead. Make a full movement of the exercise by touching the barbell to the shoulders each time it is lowered and locking the elbows each time it is pressed overhead.

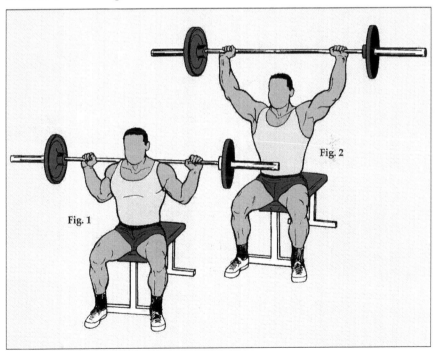

Fig. 1

Fig. 2

STANDING CHEATING SIDE LATERAL RAISE

Muscle Group: Front and outer deltoids
Degree of Difficulty: Difficult

Stand with your feet about sixteen inches apart. Grasp a dumbbell in each hand and place them in front of your thighs so your hands are facing each other and the dumbbells are touching. From this position bend slightly forward at the waist for more assistance while you start to raise the dumbbells out to the sides of the body and upward in a semicircular motion until they are a little higher than shoulder height. As you are raising the dumbbells, commence to arch your back to get a swinging effect with your upper body to help raise the dumbbells. Inhale as you raise the weights and exhale as you are lowering them. Keep your knees locked while you raise and lower the weights making the deltoids and supporting muscle groups do the bulk of the work.

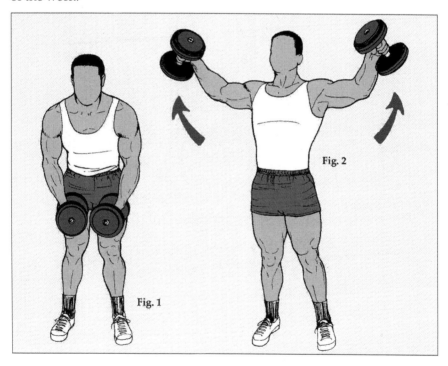

Fig. 2

Fig. 1

DUMBBELL STRAIGHT ARM FRONT DELTOID RAISE

Muscle Group: Front deltoids
Degree of Difficulty: Intermediate

Grasp a dumbbell with both hands holding them at your sides with your palms facing in, arms straight and elbows locked out. Sit at the end of a bench with your back straight and your head up. Inhale and raise both dumbbells up in a semicircular motion until they are at arm's length overhead. Lower the dumbbells back to starting position using the same semicircular motion and exhale.

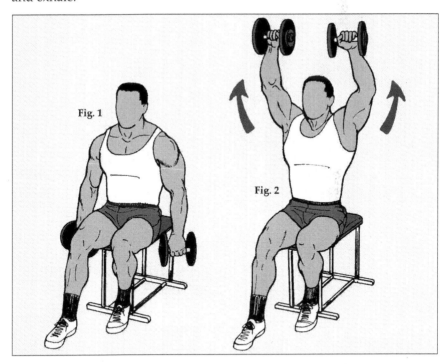

Fig. 1

Fig. 2

INCLINE DUMBBELL HELD TO THE FRONT SIDE LATERAL RAISE

Muscle Group: Rear deltoids
Degree of Difficulty: Intermediate

Lie on an incline bench with your left side on the bench. Please note the position for your feet. With a dumbbell in your right hand and placed across your body so the right hand is about even with your left thigh and your palm facing down, inhale, keeping your arm straight and elbow locked out as you raise the dumbbell in a semicircular motion straight up until it is vertical. Lower the weight in the same manner and exhale. Do the prescribed number of repetitions and then change positions, repeating the same number of repetitions with your left arm.

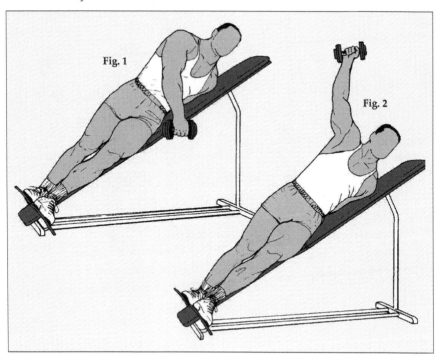

Fig. 1

Fig. 2

This page has been intentionally left blank.

Chapter 9

Course Four

The following courses are for individuals who have been training for a period of years. Beginners should do only one set of each exercise on course one. After completing the six week period, start course two and do two sets of each exercise. Do not do more than three sets of each exercise until you have been working out for a year or more. Work within your own limit

EXERCISES:

1. Standing Palm in One Arm Dumbbell Press	3 sets of 5-8
2. Incline Side Lateral Raise	3 sets of 8-10
3. Seated Barbell Military Press	4 sets of 5-8
4. Standing Alternated Front Deltoid Raise	3 sets of 8
5. Seated Side Lateral Raise	3 sets of 8

- Follow this course of exercises for a six week period
- Do Three Workouts per Week

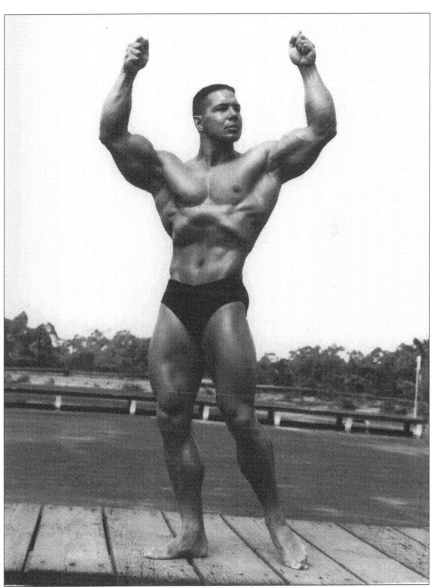

A classic pose which emphasizes the amazing difference between shoulder width and waist.

STANDING PALM IN ONE ARM DUMBBELL PRESS

Muscle Group: Front and outer deltoids
Degree of Difficulty: Intermediate

Clean a dumbbell to shoulder height. Use the other hand to hold on to an object such as an incline bench to support the upper body and lock the legs and hips solidly. Keep the elbow in slightly and have the palm of your hand facing in. Take a deep breath and press the dumbbell straight up. As you commence to lower the weight, exhale. Perform the prescribed number of repetitions and change hands. Always keep the palms facing inward.

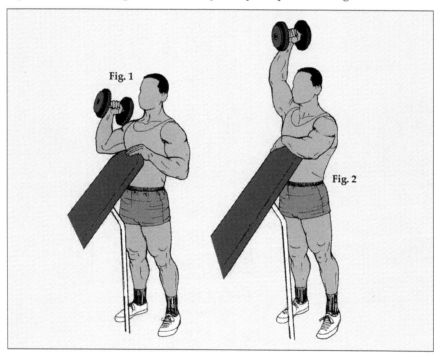

Fig. 1

Fig. 2

INCLINE SIDE LATERAL RAISE

Muscle Group: Outer deltoids
Degree of Difficulty: Intermediate

Assume the leg position on an incline bench as shown in illustration #1. Hold the dumbbell in your right hand, palm facing the thigh, raise the dumbbell to the position shown in illustration #2. Please note the position of the dumbbell. It is important to maintain the angle. Do not turn the wrist. Keep the arm straight. Inhale as you raise the dumbbell overhead, exhale as it is lowered to the thigh. Exercise the right arm and then the left.

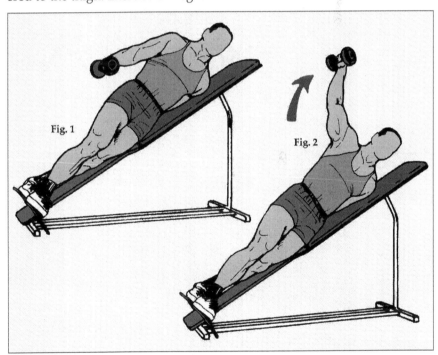

Fig. 1

Fig. 2

SEATED BARBELL MILITARY PRESS

Muscle Group: Front and outer deltoids
Degree of Difficulty: Difficult

This exercise is done exactly as a standing military press, only in a seated position, and in a stricter fashion. First, clean the barbell to the shoulders, sit down and place your feet about sixteen inches apart. Keep the chest high and your back straight. Press the barbell to arm's length overhead. Do the press slowly and steadily, keeping tension on the muscles at all times. Inhale as you push the barbell overhead and exhale as you lower the bar back to the chest.

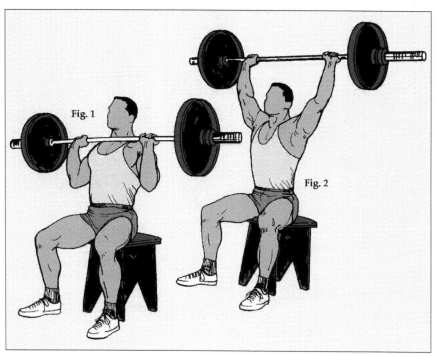

STANDING ALTERNATED FRONT DELTOID RAISE

Muscle Group: Front deltoids
Degree of Difficulty: Intermediate

Hold a dumbbell in each hand at arm's length at your sides with your palms facing toward the rear. Stand erect with your back straight, head up and hips locked. With your arms straight and your elbows locked out, raise the right dumbbell up in a semicircular motion until it is vertical. As you commence to lower the right dumbbell, start raising the left dumbbell using a similar semicircular motion so as the right dumbbell returns to starting position the left dumbbell is overhead. Inhale as you raise the right dumbbell and exhale as you raise the left dumbbell.

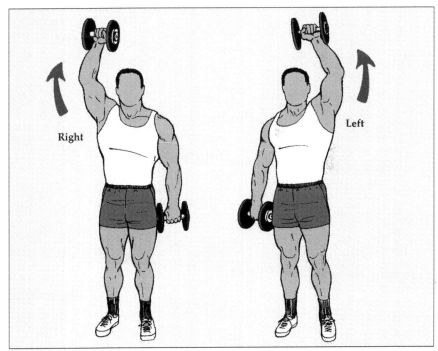

SEATED SIDE LATERAL RAISE

Muscle Group: Front and outer deltoids
Degree of Difficulty: Intermediate
Sit on the edge of a bench with your legs fairly close together and dumbbells at arm's length, palms facing in toward the thighs. Slowly raise the dumbbells to a position a little above shoulder height, pause, then lower them back to starting position. Keep the arms straight throughout the execution of the exercise. Inhale when raising the dumbbells and exhale as they are lowered.

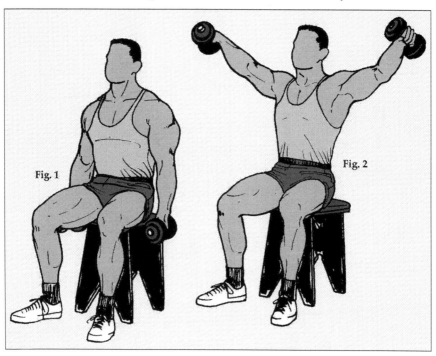

Fig. 1

Fig. 2

This page has been intentionally left blank.

Chapter 10

Course Five

The following courses are for individuals who have been training for a period of years. Beginners should do only one set of each exercise on course one. After completing the six week period, start course two and do two sets of each exercise. Do not do more than three sets of each exercise until you have been working out for a year or more. Work within your own limit

EXERCISES:

1. Seated Barbell Press in Front and Behind Neck	4 sets of 8
2. Seated Side Lateral Raise	4 sets of 8
3. Bent Over Two Dumbbell Rowing	4 sets of 8
4. Standing Dumbbell Straight Arm Front Deltoid Raise	3 sets of 6-8
5. Lying Rear Deltoid Raise	2 sets of 8-10

- Follow this course of exercises for a six week period
- Do Three Workouts per Week

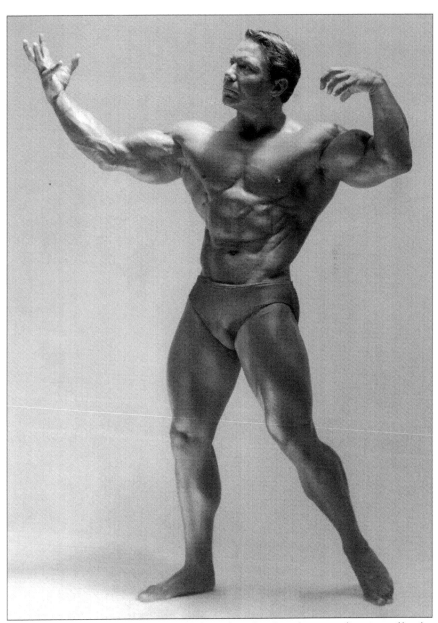

Professional Mr. Universe 1971. Bill Pearl, the end results of nearly twenty-five years of hard, continuous weight training.

SEATED BARBELL PRESS IN FRONT AND BEHIND NECK

Muscle Group: Front and outer deltoids
Degree of Difficulty: Difficult

Clean a barbell to the front of your shoulders and sit at the end of a bench. Press the barbell to arm's length overhead and then lower it behind your head to your upper back. Then press the barbell back to arm's length overhead and lower it to the front. Inhale as you are pressing and exhale as you are lowering the weight. Front and back should be considered one repetition.

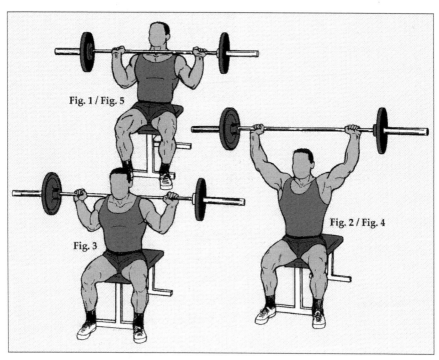

Fig. 1 / Fig. 5

Fig. 2 / Fig. 4

Fig. 3

SEATED SIDE LATERAL RAISE

Muscle Group: Front and outer deltoids
Degree of Difficulty: Intermediate
Sit on the edge of a bench with your legs fairly close together and dumbbells at arm's length, palms facing in toward the thighs. Slowly raise the dumbbells to a position a little above shoulder height, pause, then lower them back to starting position. Keep the arms straight throughout the execution of the exercise. Inhale when raising the dumbbells and exhale as they are lowered.

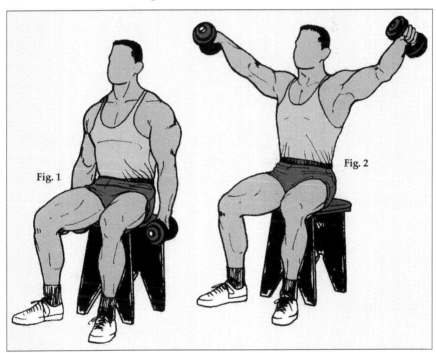

Fig. 1

Fig. 2

BENT OVER TWO DUMBBELL ROWING

Muscle Group: Lats

Degree of Difficulty: Difficult

Using a very close foot stance, place a dumbbell at each side of your feet. Bend at the waist and grasp the dumbbells with both hands with your legs slightly bent to take the pressure off your lower back. Inhale and pull both dumbbells directly up to the sides of your chest. Inhale as you pull the weights up and exhale as you let them back to starting position. Do not let the dumbbells touch the floor once you have begun the exercise. Keep your head up and your back straight.

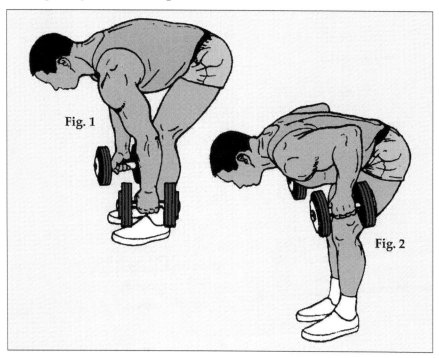

Fig. 1

Fig. 2

STANDING DUMBBELL STRAIGHT ARM FRONT DELTOID RAISE

Muscle Group: Front deltoids
Degree of Difficulty: Intermediate

Grasp a dumbbell with both hands holding either at your sides or in front of your thighs depending if you are sitting or standing. With your palms facing in, arms straight and elbows locked out, inhale and raise both dumbbells up in a semicircular motion until they are at arm's length overhead. Lower the dumbbells back to starting position using the same semicircular motion and exhale.

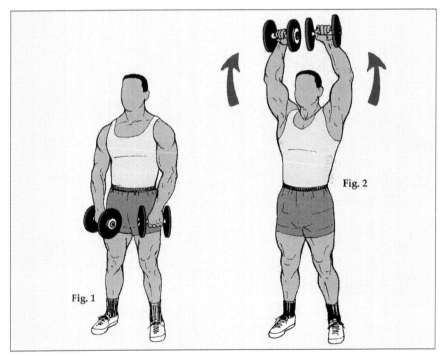

Fig. 1

Fig. 2

LYING REAR DELTOID RAISE

Muscle Group: Rear deltoids
Degree of Difficulty: Difficult

Lie face down on a fairly tall fiat bench with a dumbbell in each hand, palms facing each other. Keep your elbows locked and the arms as straight as possible as they hang straight down. Raise the dumbbells up in a semicircular motion to shoulder height. Concentrate on having your hands in line with your ears at the top of the exercise. Inhale as you raise the dumbbells and exhale as you lower them to starting position.

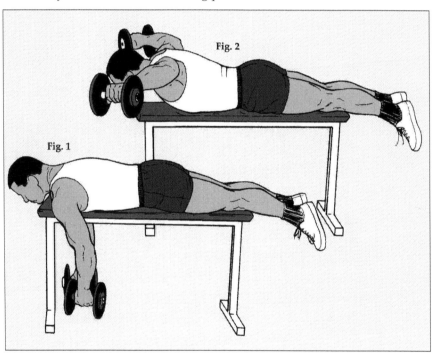

Made in the USA
San Bernardino, CA
27 July 2018